IF IT FITS YOUR MACROS

The Ultimate Flexible Diet Guidebook

Eat Whatever You Want.

Get Lean.

Lose Fat.

Connor Harper

Limit of Liability and Disclaimer of Warranty

All content in this book is provided for your information only and may not be construed as medical advice or instruction. Readers should consult appropriate health professionals on any matter relating to their health and wellbeing.

The information and opinions expressed here are believed to be accurate, based on the best judgment available to the author, and readers who fail to consult with appropriate health authorities assume the risk of any injuries.

Table of Contents

Introduction

If you are ready for a diet that works for anyone, then you have come to the right place. IIFYM (or If It Fits Your Macros) flexible dieting, is an approach that doesn't focus so much on what you eat, but on how well you balance your macronutrients. In this beginner's guide you will learn how to follow this diet whether you are used to eating organic produce or fast food. You will also learn about Body Mass Index (BMI) and how to calculate your caloric needs.

The concepts taught in this book are tried and successfully tested by many in the fitness industry. I use this method personally and endorse the concept to all my personal training clients who love it too. Your success using the IIFYM principles are largely based on self discipline and giving the diet a consistent shot at working for you. It is really an enjoyable, realistic, lifestyle change which supports both health and wellbeing goals.

Chapter 1: What is IIFYM?

IIFYM is the diet you use when you want to lose weight, but can't afford to buy organic foods, or don't have the time to eat healthy like you should. Let's face it, most of us have had days so busy that we find ourselves scarfing down McDonald's on the way to our next meeting. Well with IIFYM, you don't have to feel like you are breaking your diet to do this.

Dieting is hard. Most of us have tried and failed to stick to the regimented variety of diet plans. These plans are often confusing, expensive, and just downright time consuming if you have to prepare them yourselves. For the average person who works a nine-to-five job, this is difficult to achieve and requires a lot of discipline. The average Joe spends eight hours at work, and only has a thirty-minute lunch break. Then they have to go home, take care of the household, and make themselves a meal. Add in kids, or overtime work, and there just aren't enough hours in the day sometimes to cook regular meals, let alone follow a regimented diet plan with complex recipes.

Have you had this happen before? You start a diet plan, and you are so excited to begin. You start it on the weekend to ensure you can prepare ahead of time for the week. So you go throughout your week and eat healthy, but on Friday, you found you ran out of your pre-planned meals. So you stop and get a bite of Chinese take-out or Taco Bell, or whatever fast food you can get your hands on. You figure, no big deal, it's just one cheat day, and you will make sure to prepare better this weekend. However, you didn't take into account that it is your weekend to be Den Mother for your daughter's Girl Scout troupe, and your son has soccer practice and two birthday parties to attend. You have a dress or suit fitting to be in your best friend's wedding party and by the time you are done with everything, you realize that one cheat day turned into three, plus you don't have time to prepare for the next week, so you get discouraged and give up?

Okay so maybe it didn't happen quite like that, but I can guess that life got in the way of the perfect diet. With flexible dieting, it doesn't have to be that way. You can have a busy life, and you can eat that fast food. Just as long as you keep its nutritional value below your macronutrients cap for that meal. This is the diet for the busy person who wants to get healthy, but doesn't have the time to stick to a strict diet plan. Of course you still have to exercise, but if you have kids or an active lifestyle, you probably get plenty of that incidentally.

What is Flexible Dieting Exactly?

Despite what everyone says, science has concluded that your body does not read foods as "healthy or unhealthy", it merely takes the nutrients and substances in it and breaks it down. The only problem the body has, is that it can only break down so many values of a certain nutrient. For example, an average female body on the BMI chart (five-foot-five, one hundred and twenty pounds) should be on the standard two thousand calorie diet. This means that your body can only break down about two thousand calories a day. And based on that your body can only process a certain amount of protein, a certain amount of carbohydrates and a certain amount of fat. This value changes based on your place on the BMI scale, but the concept is still the same. Those components are called macronutrients. They are what run your body and give you the energy you need to get through the day. Each macronutrient has a specific caloric value, and it is up to you to figure out how much of each macronutrient you need to be healthy.

Everyone's body breaks macronutrients down differently. This is based on your total daily energy expenditure, or TDEE for short. Your TDEE is based on your weight and your exercise regiment. So some people may need more fat and less carbs and protein, while some require more protein than carbs and fat, and still more people need more carbs than protein and fat. Rather than tracking how many calories you eat a day, you track how many macronutrients you consume, and try to meet your daily needs on a regular basis.

How is this different than other diets, aside from tracking what you eat differently? How does this allow you to eat fast food without feeling bad? Well that is simple. A grilled chicken sandwich from McDonald's has the same macronutrients as a serving of brown rice and tuna. This means that if you have to stop at a fast food restaurant, all you have to do is check their nutritional values list for the right fit for you. Order what you want, as long as you stay within the confines of your macronutrients for the day.

You must be thinking that this is too good to be true, well I can assure you that it is not. IIFYM is the best diet out there for the average person. I have clients of diverse body types and backgrounds who have all seen great success using this methodology!

Benefits of IIFYM

There are many benefits to this diet, besides the obvious perk of losing weight. Most people are skeptical that something so easy can have results, but those results are real and there are very minimal downsides. The benefits are not to be scoffed at. Consider the below to figure out if flexible dieting is for you.

- **Sustainable:** This is a super easy diet to follow. There are no tricky recipes, no toting around your own food to places, or specific food group restrictions. Simply track what you eat. Since it is so simple to follow, a lot more people find that they stick with it. Especially since it means they don't have to give up the foods they love. It is also an easy diet to expand upon. You can start out just trying to meet your macronutrients, and then once you achieve and sustain this, you can try to eat healthier foods to meet your macronutrients and ensure you are getting essential vitamins, minerals, and fiber in your diet. Because you are already used to tracking your food, it will be easy to just add a few more things to monitor.

  It's also a super sustainable diet due to the fact that if you do fall off the wagon for a day, you don't have a whole load of prep-work to do to get back on your diet. You just track your macros the next day, and continue on as if nothing ever happened. That is an awesome thing to be able to do. You can have a cheat day without feeling super guilty which is not something you can say about most diets. That guilt free ease in which you can eat food is what makes this diet sustainable.

- **No Tupperware:** When you were on other diets, how often did you bring your own container of food to a dinner party so you wouldn't have to cheat on your diet in a social setting? It gets kind of awkward when everyone else is having barbequed chicken, and you are in the back by yourself eating cold rice and tuna. Or worse so, sitting there while everyone is enjoying Mexican food, and you are drinking a kale smoothie all the while being taunted by the delicious smells wafting under your nose.

It can also be awkward for those around you as well. They want to ask about your diet, but are afraid to offend you. The fact of the matter is that most diets are not conducive to a social atmosphere, so they are not suited to the average lifestyle.

With flexible dieting, you don't have to bring your own food already prepared, and you can join in with what everyone else is having, just track the food, track what you ate, and ask for the recipe so you can look it up online later. This leaves you able to socialize without awkward stares and feeling left out as everyone enjoys food you are forbidden to eat. Go ahead. Eat the cake, and do so without a shred of guilt. Just remember that moderation is key.

- **No Confusing Recipes:** You don't have to be a great chef with a diverse repertoire of clean recipes to follow this diet either. Most diets out there require cooking skills, but with flexible dieting, what you normally eat will suffice. Just cut your portions to match your macros. You don't need to know what a chia seed is, or how to make an eggplant puree, just know the nutritional values of what you cook and you are all set.

There are many tools and apps out there that can help you track what you eat, so there is less stress on you. You can input your meal and look up nutritional values as well, making flexible dieting even easier. You can also use these tools to get recipes ideas to make your macros stretch farther, that way you feel more full. Instead of having to arrange a grocery list a mile long, you can get your normal essentials, and call it good.

- **No Extensive Prep-work:** Many diets require you to make your meals in advance and freeze them for the week to ensure you can stick to a plan. This approach requires the discipline to reserve cooking time on a regular basis. You also have to figure out just how many meals you need, and what meals you want for what days. After that you have to compile a grocery list and make sure you have everything. Then you spend the greater part of the weekend cooking foods you don't even really like before forcing yourself to eat them through the week. Doesn't seem very fun, does it?

With IIFYM, you don't have to do all that prep-work. Don't have time to cook breakfast? Grab a bagel on your way out the door. There is no requirement to eat anything specific, and you don't have to waste your weekends shopping and cooking. This diet is a breeze, and there is no denying that easy is the best policy when it comes to dieting.

Are you still skeptical? These benefits alone are enough to outshine most other diets, but there are a few more that you should know about in case you are not yet convinced.

- **No Fasting:** Many diets require a fast or cleanse of some sort, or abstinence from eating at certain times. This often requires consuming nothing but juices or liquids such as green tea, or some sort of kale smoothie. These approaches are off putting and leave you hungry or dissatisfied a lot of the time. Fasting can also be harmful for your metabolism, shifting it into survival mode and effectively slowing down your ability to digest food.

  IIFYM does not require a fast of any sort. Nor do you have to do an uncomfortable colon cleanse. You do not have to make dramatic habit changes and have the luxury of being yourself with no negative implication on your metabolism.

- **No Miracle Foods, No Fees:** Flexible dieting embodies the belief that there are no miracle or fad super foods. All food options can get you to your goal weight without having to buy some expensive product. There are also no fees to join a group that will teach you about counting calories, and you don't have to buy some pricey pyramid scheme weight loss product that doesn't work, yet it lures you in with photo-shopped or misleading pictures of results. You don't have to spend upwards of eighty dollars a month, and have to follow a rigorous diet and exercise regime. Your body does not need a hyped shake product or skinny tea plan to lose weight.

  You also don't have to eat a bunch of kale and spinach to follow this diet. You can eat tasty food if you so desire, and it will not produce poor physical results. You are still staying in the confines of your macros and that is what this diet is all about.

- **Not Just for Weight Loss:** The great thing about this diet is that it is versatile. You don't just have to use it to lose weight. If you are trying to improve your body structure or composition, you can use this diet to do so as well. Just change your macros up a bit. If you want more muscle, eat more protein. If you want less muscle, eat less protein. If you want to gain weight due to being on the thin side, then add more carbs and fats to meet a higher caloric value. IIFYM is an approach that is very adaptable and known as flexible dieting for this reason.

They don't lie when they say that this is the diet for everyone. It is so easy to adapt to your needs, and it doesn't involve anything extra to use to change. You simply switch up how you track your macros.

- **Be Present:** The best part about this diet is that it allows you to actively be a part of your life, without the constraints of a diet. You don't have to run home in the middle of your son's soccer game because you forgot to take your supplement. You don't have to carry whole grain snacks with you to eat while everyone else is eating hearty sandwiches. You don't have to miss your daughter's ballet recital because you are too busy doing your week's worth of meal prep that day.

You can be present in the moment, and really enjoy the people around you without feeling guilty about having a burger at a cookout. You can enjoy every joke, every smile, every laugh, without having to excuse yourself to go eat your food away from everyone else to avoid the awkwardness. You can join everyone else at the table and enjoy the food along with your friends. I know that IIFYM has made a big difference to my life personally, and this is why I want to share my passion for the approach.

Hopefully by now these benefits are enough to convince you that flexible dieting is for anyone, and you can start your journey to a new you. Everyone deserves a diet that allows them the freedoms of life. If you live a busy lifestyle, you may use the excuse "oh I just don't have time to track what I eat." However, there are tools out there to help you, and most are free. So there really is no excuse not to try this approach for yourself.

Continue reading to learn more about IIFYM and figure out if it is right for you. This chapter will contain more information on what macros are, and what you need to know about the origin of macros.

Macronutrients, what are they exactly?

Macronutrients are the nutrients that your body needs to turn food into energy. These are often portrayed in three groups: fat, protein, and carbohydrates. These nutrients are the most important part of meeting your caloric intake for weight loss. Each of these nutrients also contain sub categories. For example, oils are considered a part of the fat category, and sugars are part of the carbohydrate category, and so on and so forth. Every nutrient also has a caloric value. That is what makes them so important. Rather than the ever-followed fad of counting this value, you are counting the nutrient that make up the calories. This ensures that you are balanced on the types of calories you need for your body structure.

At first glance this may seem needlessly complicated. Why count three different things when I can count just one? The answer is that by emphasizing specific amounts of each macronutrient (and choosing quality sources), you can better tailor it to your lifestyle, tastes, and physical goals.

Origins of Flexible Dieting

The IIFYM concept started out as an insider tactic used by bodybuilders, rather than by people wanting to lose weight. These bodybuilders wanted to know if they could eat other things rather than just what qualified as competition prep food, due to dietary restrictions. This started the phrase, 'if it fits your macros, go ahead and eat it'. It got tiresome to write out over and over, and then the phrase IIFYM was born. This approach quickly gained in popularity and then spread to other areas of dieting, and after a phase of experimentation it was found to be a very versatile diet plan. Thus flexible dieting became the diet for everyone.

The Difference Between Fat Loss and Weight Loss

In traditional dieting, the goal is merely weight loss, not fat loss. Your goal is to shed as many pounds as you can, no matter what you lose. In most of these diets, the pounds you lose are water weight pounds. This means that you still have the fat on your body, you are just less water. Also with diets that require a fast or cleanse, you may be losing muscle as well, so while the number is going down on the scale, you are not getting any healthier, as most of your fat is still in place. Tracking your macros allows you to use your BMI to deduce how many macronutrients you need to help your body break down the fat stores it has, and become healthier, not just skinnier on the scales.

The true goal in dieting should be losing as many pounds of fat as possible. Fat clogs your arteries and raises your cholesterol level. The higher the fat content is in your body, the higher the risk becomes of you developing coronary problems. You don't need to avoid certain foods to remove this fat from your body either. You merely have to cut down your portions of certain foods. Once you figure out exactly how many macros you need, you can begin losing fat. Then you can become a healthier you.

In the next chapters you will learn all the basics of following IIFYM. This includes calculating your total daily energy expenditure, and how to figure out within those confines what grams of each macro you need to reach your goal. You will also learn about different foods you can eat to get the most out of your macros, and the common pitfalls of this diet, that way you can avoid them and be a success.

Chapter 2: Flexible Dieting Vs Standard Dieting

Avoiding the "OFF-LIMITS" Stigma

With regular diets there is generally an extensive list of foods you are not able to eat. Most lists consist of anything processed, which let's face it, is anything not in the fresh produce aisle at the grocery store. This does not make for a very happy dieter, and an unhappy dieter is not going to commit to the diet for very long.

With flexible dieting, there is no prohibited list of foods that you cannot eat. There is no need to throw out half of the food in your pantry. You can keep everything you normally consume, just work on portion control. You don't have to have a new list of foods in your fridge, and you don't need to eat a diet that makes you gag or dread mealtimes.

While this does not mean that you can live off of junk food, the occasional donut is not a death sentence to your diet. The idea is to still eat healthy food, but you don't have to give up your guilty pleasures to follow the diet. You can have a processed snack once in a while or stop by the drive through on a busy day and not have to count it as a cheat day.

The stigma that some foods should be avoided comes from the belief that anything processed has chemicals that cause illness and are carcinogenic, and that you should not consume them for your wellbeing. It originally had nothing to do with losing weight. Since then people have been on these clean binges and of course, as they are not putting anything with fat content in their bodies they are losing weight, but is it really healthy?

How Healthy is 'Clean Eating' Really?

Everyone says that clean eating is the way to go, and clean eating can be great if done right. However, most people do not go about clean eating the right way, and if done wrong, it can have seriously unhealthy effects on your metabolism.

As stated before, most diets that involve clean eating also involve a fast of some sort. Sometimes they are called colon cleanses. During these fasts you are not allowed to eat anything, and have to consume unpalatable drinks that clear out all of the "toxins" in your colon. These drinks often contain very little nutritional value, and do not give you the nutrients you need to sustain your metabolism. So if you are following these fasts, they generally last for up to two weeks. That is two weeks that your metabolism has nothing to run on.

As with diets where you are starving yourself, fasting hurts your metabolism severely. If you do it once, you may not have any effects if you are lucky, but if you do it regularly, your metabolism will definitely be impacted. This can cause your body to shift into survival mode and convert every bit of food it receives into fat stores. Over time, no matter what you eat, you will not be able to easily lose weight.

Clean eating even without fasting can be damaging. Whilst consuming a range of wholefoods is something we recommend, people can inadvertently cut out essential nutrients by avoiding entire food groups. This is particularly common when undertaking a vegan diet without a proper assessment of foods consumed and their underlying macronutrients.

The problem lies with getting the starches and carbohydrates you need from foods other than potatoes. Unless you make your own pasta or bread, you are going to have to buy store bought varieties. There are many other things that your body needs due to the fat content, and if you are avoiding these foods, you may become malnourished. This is the problem a lot of clean eating dieters do not understand. You have to make sure that you are getting the necessary nutrients to support your metabolism. After your metabolism crashes, your thyroid is next, and it is all downhill from there.

An uninformed clean eater can do more harm than good. All they are doing is starving their body so that it eats fat stores, and causes muscle mass to deteriorate. This is not healthy, and can result in some major damage to the system.

With flexible dieting, it doesn't matter if you eat organic or processed foods. All that matters is that you eat foods that meet your macros standards. You don't run the risk of harming your metabolism, and don't have to strain your budget by buying all new groceries. You can eat foods that have all the vitamins and minerals you need, with no threat of malnutrition. Well, as long as you don't try to survive on junk food.

There are No Good or Bad Foods

I know your entire life you have been lead to believe that certain foods are bad for you and that you should never eat them. This is the farthest from the truth. The body does not interpret food as healthy or unhealthy. It merely sees the food you are eating as nutrients to break down and use, and then it stores what it cannot use as fat deposits. The goal is to use up all the nutrients in your food so none has to be stored.

You are probably wondering how this is done, if you can eat anything you desire. The answer is simple. Portion control. This is the key to weight loss. Most people eat twice as much as their body needs to sustain itself, and all that extra food has to go somewhere, and that somewhere is the fat deposits on the human body. To avoid these fat deposits, you merely figure out how much food you need to break down along with your energy expenditure, and consume no more than that. You need only enough to meet your daily needs. Do not exceed them.

In this day and age, it seems impossible to get that satiated full feeling when you only meet the amount of food you need to eat. The portions provided in restaurants and take-out meals well exceed that required by your body in one meal setting. In reality, you are not supposed to be full when you finish eating. That room left over should be filled with water. Over eighty percent of people do not drink enough water daily. You should be drinking a gallon of water every day. It seems like a lot, but in reality it isn't. There are eight cups in a gallon, and most people are awake for sixteen hours a day. That is one cup every two hours. Broken up like that, it seems a lot easier to manage. If you drink plenty of water, then only consuming the amount of macros you need becomes a lot easier.

Any food can be used to lose weight, as long as you are getting a balanced diet with all the nutrients required to maintain proper nutrition. Ensure that you consume plenty of iron and fiber, and don't overdo the sugar intake, so your insulin can handle it.

If you think back on prior occasions where you have restricted yourself, it is likely to have been a bad idea because it always backfires. You stay away from chocolate, and ignore it in the grocery store, but the cravings don't go away. How many times while on a diet did you avoid your favorite food, and you were doing really good for a while, and didn't stand in front of the shelf before forcing yourself to walk away without it? How long did that go on before you had a really bad day and all of a sudden you were binging on that delicious food, eating way more than you should? A week? A month? When you restrict yourself, eventually you are going to snap, and over consume the food you were trying to stay away from. Then you end up eating way more than a healthy amount. However, if you merely cut down the portions of how much you eat, then you will still be satisfied, and less likely to binge later.

Along with the physical effects of binging, research studies have found that people following a restrictive approach to dieting were more likely to have a higher BMI, reduced feelings of self-control, and more psychological stress related to weight and food intake. Traditional dieting can be just as taxing on mental wellbeing as it is on your body.

Many studies on the IIFYM diet have been undertaken, and people have sworn by it in the wider fitness community. Dr. Layne Norton (2012) has done extensive research on the diet by studying bodybuilders and how well this approach helped them. He monitored a group of bodybuilders who only ate clean food, and then monitored a group that followed IIFYM principles. The IIFYM group saw more success in hitting their goals, because they did not end up binging on their favorite foods, as they never had to quit eating them. A key finding was that this avoidance of cheat days greatly enhanced dieting success. If you want something, you fit it into your macros. Simple as that.

The study also also discussed how many coaches used the IIFYM method to ensure that their wrestlers and bodybuilders can meet their weight goals, and be in the right bracket during a competition. They do not have to worry about their athletes sneaking in a meal that will throw their entire diet off, because there are no foods that are considered off limits with flexible dieting.

Chapter 3: Macros and How to Track Them

Macros 101

As stated above, macronutrients are an essential part of your everyday life. These nutrients are what give you energy, and allow your metabolism to function properly. Without the right amount of certain macros, you will find you probably have trouble losing weight. Macronutrients all have a caloric value, but rather than just tracking calories, you track the nutrients that make up those calories. This ensures you have the right ones for your body structure, because if you don't have the correct types of calories, you may not be giving your body the proper nutrition it needs to function at its best. Everyone's body is different, so they have to track their macros differently. This is why calorie counting diets never work. You can't just eat anything that falls within your calorie limit, because you may be getting too much of one macronutrient, but not enough of the others.

Macros are broken down into three categories. These categories are as follows:

- **Fat:** Yes, fat is a necessary part of a normal diet. There are actual fats that are good for you and essential for a healthy diet. You do not want to shy away from consuming these as your metabolism will not be able to function, because this is the driving force behind a well tuned body. Fat is used and turned into energy. This energy is used to regulate your hormones, form cell membranes, and improve brain function. These fats also help to give you healthy skin, hair, and nails. They aid in the regulation of temperature and carry vitamins throughout your body as well. There are four types of fats:

  Monounsaturated Fat: These fats are good for your heart, and help to decrease the level of unhealthy fat in your bloodstream. There are several foods that you can eat that contain a healthy amount of these fats. These include avocados, olive oil, peanut butter, and almonds.

  Polyunsaturated Fat: These fats are necessary to for healthy brain function, skin and hair growth, prevention of heart attacks, and control of blood pressure and clotting. There are two categories of polyunsaturated fats – linoleic (omega-6) and linolenic (omega-3). These essential fats cannot be produced from other fats in your body and must be obtained through your diet. You can find them in foods like salmon, tuna, nuts, seeds and soybean oil.

Saturated Fat: These fats are also known as animal fats because they are contained in in many meat and dairy products, such as milk, cheese, butter, and cream. Consumption of these fats in your diet should be limited. Too much can raise your cholesterol and cause negative health implications for your heart and blood pressure.

Trans Fat: These are the unhealthiest of fats, and should only be consumed in minute doses. These fats severely increase levels of bad cholesterol and can lead to the clogging of your arteries. They are found in many processed foods such as margarine, deep-fried take-outs and baked goods like biscuits, cakes and pastries.

Those are the four types of fats and how they affect you. Remember, unsaturated fats are best, and trans fats are the worst. If you monitor your fat intake well, you should be able to maintain maximum health.

- **Carbohydrates:** Contrary to many misleading diet claims, carbs are not the enemy. They are an important component of your everyday diet. These are broken down into energy used to digest food, and also create enzymes in the small intestine that allow you to pass out all waste without getting ill. Carbohydrates comprise of five forms:

  Monosaccharides: These simple sugars form the most basic units of carbohydrates. They are also known as glucose or fructose, and are found in many natural foods, such as berries, honey, and syrups or nectars. Monosaccharides are a water soluble sugar that sweeten these foods naturally, and give them a golden brown color when reduced.

  Disaccharides: Also known as sucrose, it is a substance that acts as a natural sweetener in foods. It can be in crystal or liquid form, and is found in many natural foods. Lactose, found in milk, is also considered to be a disaccharide. Lactose is what gives milk its sweet taste, and can be an allergen for some individuals.

Oligosaccharides: Do not occur very frequently in foods. This form of carbohydrate serves as added fiber and have a probiotic function. Found in foods such as onions, lentils and beans, they contain the enzymes that convert into fecal matter through the waste process.

Polysaccharides: Or starches, are the most abundant of carbohydrates that are out there. Many people associate carbs with starchy foods, rather than veggies and fruits. You have been told that these foods are bad, but that is quite the opposite. Starches are one of the most important components of your diet as they help to absorb nutrients into the bloodstream. Polysaccharides are contained in foods such as wheat, oats, rye, barley, potatoes and legumes.

- **Protein:** This forms one of the most essential elements to our diet, as it is what builds muscle and allows it to heal after injury. It also contains a lot of iron, which helps to regulate your blood composition, and prevents you from becoming anemic.

Protein is formed from a combination of twenty amino acids. There are nine essential amino acids (cannot be made by the body and must be sourced through your diet) and eleven non-essential amino acids which your body is able to produce. All of these acids are necessary to thrive, but the amount in which they need to be present varies. Protein allows you to have a strong and healthy body, and that is the goal of any diet. Being healthy will allow you to live life to the fullest, without always being sluggish and tired.

Essential amino acids are contained in foods such as eggs, animal proteins, quinoa, soy and kidney beans. Supplementation of non-essential amino acids in the body can be done through consuming whole foods like nuts, grains, meats, fruits and vegetables.

Macronutrients Breakdown

Most dieticians say you should have a 40/30/30 diet when breaking down macros. This means forty percent protein, thirty percent fat, and thirty percent carbs. However, this concept has been superseded by the block diet theory (e.g. Zone and Paleo). This approach extols that individuals require more carbohydrates than protein. This has been the style that athletes adhere to religiously as it is seen to produce the best results.

The framework for this breakdown is for every pound you weigh, you need between 0.5 and 1 gram of protein depending on your activity level. And for every seven grams of protein you require, you need nine grams of carbs and three grams of fats.

Tracking

You can track your macros by looking up the nutritional information online and then noting them down. This is the way a lot of old-school athletes do it. However, you can also use a handy phone app or go online to resources such as myfitnesspal.com, a website that will help you track your macros, and even look up nutritional info for you.

Why You Should Track

You should track what you eat, that way you can be sure that you are meeting your nutritional requirements. For those with busy lifestyles, it helps to time when you last ate to ensure your mealtimes are balanced. This will serve to call out instances of late night binging and promote a habit of regular eating for optimum body metabolism. Get a little planner and use it to write down what you consume each day, and to keep track of its macronutrient value.

Tracking the types of foods you consume will also enable you to see the progress you have made in cleaning up your diet, as well as how you have improved in splitting your macros up evenly without going over or under. The more validation you have of your progress, the more you will want to align to the flexible dieting methodology for ultimate success.

The main advantage of tracking your macros, specifically, is that you can optimize the ratios for your specific body needs. For example, if you are doing high intensity exercise and weight training, then you can maximize results by increasing your carbohydrate intake. Your body may also respond better by reducing your fat intake slightly to compensate for the added carbs, leading to better performance and muscle definition.

Remember, each person has a different baseline of metabolism and body function. It may take a month or so of tweaking your ratios to find what works optimally for your specific bodily needs.

Do I Need to Track with 100% Accuracy?

Unless you are a hard-core body builder, tracking with total accuracy is not a requirement. Flexible dieting allows you to consume foods within 10 grams of your target protein and carbohydrate intake. For example, if your goal is 300 grams of carbohydrates, then anything from 290 to 310 grams is fine. The net difference in calories is negligible and will not negatively impact your diet results. Often the breakdown of restaurant foods and take-outs may be slightly off, so this buffer provides some relief from over analysis of each meal.

Conversely, you should take slightly more caution when consuming fats as they contain double the calories of protein and carbs. Ensure that you keep your fat intake within a 5 gram fluctuation of your goal intake. If your aim is to eat only 50 grams of fat a day, then anywhere between 45 to 55 grams will be okay. That being said, do not stress over exact macros, just try to come within a small deviation of your target. Your body does not detect perfect macros so there is no point in getting them absolutely right. Stressing out about eating perfectly can actually be counterproductive to your physique goals, so don't freak out if you miss your macros every now and then!

Working Out Your Macronutrient Ratio

There are a number of steps required to assess what percentage split is needed in each macros category. As an initial step, you need to calculate your base metabolic rate and consider this in line with your body goals. This information will then enable you to determine whether you need to adjust your daily caloric intake.

Step 1: Calculate your daily caloric intake
In order to find your caloric intake, you need to find your base metabolic rate (BMR) and your total daily energy expenditure (TDEE).

Female BMR = 655 + (4.35 x weight in pounds) + (4.7 x height in inches) - (4.7 x age in years)
Male BMR = 66 + (6.23 x weight in pounds) + (12.7 x height in inches) - (6.8 x age in years)

To find your TDEE, input your BMR into the below equation based on how active you are:

- **Sedentary** = BMR X 1.2 (little or no exercise, desk job)
- **Lightly active** = BMR X 1.375 (light exercise/sports 1-3 days/week)
- **Moderately active** = BMR X 1.55 (moderate exercise/sports 3-5 days/week)
- **Very active** = BMR X 1.725 (hard exercise/sports 6-7 days/week)
- **Extremely active** = BMR X 1.9 (hard daily exercise/sports & physical job)

This new number is your estimated daily caloric intake in kilocalories (kcal).

*Alternatively, there are many free online calculators which will work out your daily caloric intake for you.

Step 2: Define your body goals

Are you looking into flexible dieting to improve overall health? Are you happy with your current weight? Would you like to improve your body composition so that the amount of body fat to muscle decreases? Simply put, if you want to lose weight, you will need to decrease your caloric intake and conversely so if you would like to gain weight.

Regardless of whether you're trying to lose or gain pounds, your goal should be to aim for no more than a one percent change of body weight per week. This is a guideline which enables a healthy and optimal change to your body composition. For example, a man who is 180 pounds and wants to lose weight will set a goal of 1.8 pounds' reduction per week. Any more and it may adversely impact muscle loss and induce a slowing of your metabolism.

The amount of calories you consume daily is the key nutritional metric to consider when it comes to gaining or losing weight. The total amount of calories you eat in a day is made of the macronutrient types we defined earlier: fats, carbohydrates and protein.

Sample Calculation:
A moderately active 30 year old woman, 160lb, 5ft 5in, has a goal of losing weight in a sustainable manner.

BMR = 1,425 kcal. TDEE = 1,425 kcal/day * 1.55 = 2,209 kcal/day

Using this current daily caloric intake, the woman is able to tailor her target caloric intake based on body goals:

Losing weight: Reduce food consumption by 500 kcal per day. She should then consume 2,209 – 500 = <u>1,709 kcal</u> daily to yield a healthy 1lb loss in body weight per week.

Step 3: Determine your protein intake

The amount of protein your body requires is based on the amount of muscle mass that you have. The way in which you use your muscle mass will also influence the quantity of this macronutrient required. For example, if you undertake regular weight training, you probably require more dietary protein than someone who focuses on cardio based exercises.

As a baseline, individuals should consume at least 0.8 grams of protein per per pound of body weight.

Body Weight (lb) x 0.8 = **Recommended daily amount (RDA) of Protein**

Note that if your RDA of protein is significantly higher than what you are currently consuming then consider gradually increasing your intake. A sudden spike of protein in your diet may cause stomach issues and will take time for your body to adjust. Adding 15 to 20 grams of protein a week is a good target to have which will not cause too much stress on your digestive system.

Step 4: Determine your fat intake

Consuming a balance of good fats (polyunsaturated and monounsaturated) daily is important for a variety of bodily functions. However, too much dietary fat can also result in adverse health consequences. To ensure that you have calculated the optimum proportion of fat, it is necessary to consider your body type and the way in which it utilizes this macronutrient. Most individuals will fit into the following categories, use this to assess your type and substitute your total daily energy expenditure into the equations:

Ectomorph: Characterized by a delicate build, they are naturally slim and often find it hard to gain weight due to a fast metabolism. Their hips and shoulders are approximately the same width, with long arms and legs. Ectomorphs typically don't require as much fat - about 25% on a daily basis.

TDEE x .25 = RDA of Fat (kcal)
Divide above RDA (kcal) by 9 = **RDA Fat in grams**

Endomorph: A naturally heavier individual, with a curvy body and larger bones. They hold fat deposits mainly in the hips, abdomen and thighs, and tend to put on weight easily. Endomorphs typically require about 35% of fat in their daily diet intake.

TDEE x .35 = RDA for Fat (kcal)
Divide above RDA (kcal) by 9 = **RDA Fat in grams**

Mesomorph: Tend to have the most proportionate of body types and is the average between endomorphs and ectomorphs in daily fat requirements. Mesomorphs store fat evenly throughout their bodies, have taut stomachs, and are able to gain muscle quickly.

TDEE x .3 = RDA for Fat (kcal)
Divide above RDA (kcal) by 9 = **RDA Fat in grams**

Step 5: Determine your carbohydrate intake
Now that you have your ideal daily protein and fat intake, use these figures to calculate your rate of carbohydrate consumption in the below equation:

TDEE – Protein calories – Fat calories = **RDA for Carbohydrates**

Now that you have your Macronutrient Ratio...

If you stick to your calculated split and commit to regular exercise, these macros will enable you to meet your body or weight loss goals for the next 6 to 8 weeks. At this point, check in on your progression and lower or adjust the ratio accordingly. Ensure that you give your body enough time to normalize on this eating regime before changing around your consumption. There is no optimal or "right" macro split. Remember, each person has a different natural metabolism and rate of body function. It may take a period of time to tweak your ratio to find what works optimally for your specific body. As you become more experienced in IIFYM methodology, the more intuitive you are about how your body responds to certain levels of macros.

Should my Macronutrient Ratio be the same every day?

From a physiological perspective, a person on the IIFYM diet should adjust their macros for days during which they are exercising or training. For example, if your ratio requires the consumption of 150 grams of carbohydrates daily, you may opt to increase this to 280 grams on a day where you are hitting the gym. If you choose not to adjust (as sometimes your meals are already prepped for ease of tracking), you may find that you hit your body goals sooner, and thus may compensate for this when reviewing your macros split over time. This really depends on your capacity to judge accurate macros and whether you are committed to a slightly more variable eating regime.

If you prefer to differentiate for training days, ensure that the level of fats and protein consumed are kept consistent. Review the amount of carbohydrates expended for your particular form of exercise and add this to your meal plan.

Should I compensate for remaining calories?

Once you have hit your macros split for the day, people often find that they have not met their calculated calorie intake. Don't worry too much about this as it is a common occurrence when undertaking flexible dieting. Over time, the diversity of food options that you consume tends to balance out any caloric deficits. In practice, this means that today's slight deficit will compensate for tomorrow's slight excess. Trying to fill in the remaining calories will throw off your macros split for the day and make the diet much more difficult to practice. Focus on achieving your ratio and the rest will even out during the week.

Chapter 4: How to Succeed on this Diet

Just like with any diet, you want to succeed, right? Are you scared that this diet will flop like all the others, and you will end up feeling like a failure, binging on processed foods while watching TV reruns to feel better? Are you worried about the diet failing?

This chapter is all about turning your diet into a success, so that you finally have that ability to balance good eating principles along with a busy lifestyle, and maybe even coach your friends to success as well. These tips are created to motivate you and warn you of mistakes to avoid, so that you don't fall off the wagon. While it is a pretty easy diet, it is still easy to get discouraged, and that is the enemy to any diet. I hope this motivates you in the way that you need, and gives you everything you need to succeed.

Have the Right Mindset

You can't go into this diet being skeptical about it. You have to believe it will work, that way you can stick with it, and know that you are doing a good job. You also have to want to do it. You will not see astounding results immediately, as with any diet. It is unreasonable to expect a miracle to happen overnight. IIFYM is a sustainable, gradual and safe way to progress towards your body goals.

As with any diet, you have to be willing to work for it. You have to be willing to exercise, and you have to be willing to put forth an effort to get the results that you are looking for.

You do not have to be a world class athlete or bodybuilder to have this mindset either. You merely have to want to succeed, and do whatever it takes to stick with it and make it. This diet is easier to commit to than most others, but it still takes patience as you struggle to reach your goal and incorporate tracking macros as a firm habit.

As with anything, it takes a bit of time to see results. Be reasonable with your goals and the timelines to achieve them. You can't expect to lose twenty pounds in one week, so don't beat yourself up for not losing fifty pounds in a month. Always give yourself a realistic time frame to reach a goal such as twenty pounds a month. This is an ambitious aim, but not a ridiculous one.

You also have to have the mindset that this is not a regular diet. Undo the years of conditioning from other diet fads and meal plans where you were told to avoid specific foods. Don't tell yourself you can't have a food because it is not healthy. That is the whole point of flexible dieting and IIFYM. To be able to eat the foods other diets say you can't. If you remember that you can eat what you want, so long as you control the portions, you will be able to go farther in this diet than you ever thought possible.

This is not just a diet, this can be a lifestyle choice. How nice would it be to not have to constantly diet after every holiday? To be able to partake in holiday food without a shred of guilt as to what it is going to do to your diet? Make macros a part of your life, and they will suit you well. While everyone else is dieting, you can sit back while eating a cupcake, and enjoy.

Don't fall into the trap others like to set for people who go against the norm. Ignore the skepticism from others who say that this diet won't work and assess for yourself, because it absolutely does. Keep your head up, and you will be able to sustain IIFYM concepts well.

Challenge Yourself

Boredom is your worst enemy in a diet. If you do the same thing over and over, you will become complacent. This is not a good thing, because once you become complacent, it is all downhill from there. You begin to cheat a little bit, and you start going over your macros, because you forget to track them. Do not allow yourself to get bored.

To avoid this problem, you can set mini goals that are a little harder to reach and try to meet them. The extra ambition it will take will help push you onwards towards your goal. This gives you something extra to work for, and makes the diet exciting again. There are several mini goals you can set such as:

- Trying to eat home cooked meals all week: While IIFYM allows you to be able to eat fast food, these options are often high in trans fat, which is not easily broken down in your body and is bad for your cholesterol levels. Home cooked meals are less likely to have high levels of trans fat, sugar and additives.

- Try to fill a day's worth of macros with a food of every color: Pick one day to do this, and that day try to fill your limit with foods that correspond to every color of the rainbow (i.e. strawberries, oranges, squash, spinach, blueberries, blackberries, and plums). This will diversity the range of vitamins and nutrients that you consume for overall wellbeing.

- Try to meet your macros while eating out at a restaurant... without using a nutritional value calculator: Review the menu and find foods that you would eat to fulfill your daily macros entirely, and write them down. Estimate the number of each macronutrient in the dishes, and then after you have played this guessing game, you can finally use a nutritional value calculator to see if you were right. Over time you will be able to memorize macro values for certain dishes and this will make flexible dieting that much easier.

- Switch up your usual menu: Look for new recipes to try with your favorite foods. This will give you a little more variety and spice up your diet. Remember that avoiding the monotony of chicken and broccoli each day is a key benefit of flexible dieting, so take advantage of it!

- Another way to avoid being bored is to try to get a few friends to join you in the flexible dieting world. This way you can share tips, and get ideas on what new foods to try. It is always easier to enjoy something when you don't feel alone. And if you have friends who are also part of the IIFYM community, they can help remind you to track what you eat, and you can do the same for them.

- There are also online forums for IIFYM on Facebook and fitness websites. You can join these to talk to people, scour the comments for tips, and get advice on how you should go about starting. These forums can be really fun and interesting. You get to talk to people from around the world who are on the same diet as you, and be motivated by seeing the real-life results of others.

There are many things you can do to avoid complacency in your dieting. Try the tips above, and see if you can come up with some ideas of your own. The more ways you have to switch things up and make them interesting, the better chance you have at being successful at this diet for the long term.

Plan Your Meals

This is not a necessity, but a good approach to take if you are the organized type. This doesn't mean you have to stick strictly to the meals as they are planned, it is just to give you a better chance of meeting your macros accurately. There are several ways in which you can plan your meals.

You can look up recipes and foods which align to your required macros online, and decide which weeks you want to do what meals. This is a good idea, because it is not giving you a specific date you have to eat that meal, which confines the diet and makes it less flexible. It also gives you a little goal to meet to make things fun. Try to squeeze all that week's meals in without leaving one out.

You can also pre plan thirty meals, and do the grocery shopping for the month to ensure that you have all the ingredients. I call this expert mode. This is after you have gotten a feel for your months, and what days you are too busy to eat a planned meal on. Once you get a sense for that you can make a goal to eat all the prepped meals in one month without leaving any out. This can be challenging and fun. It can also stave off dietary boredom.

Or you can plan out each meal for every day. This severely limits the flexibility of the diet, and should only be used if you feel you have to have the rigidity of a normal diet to reach success. And some people do need that structure. So this would be a great idea for those individuals. However, this is a diet based on flexibility, which is what draws people to IIFYM principles, so the rigid type personalities are few and far between.

Track Your Progress:

Sometimes it is hard to see just how far you have come by looking in the mirror. Our brains still see us as the same person we were. This can make it discouraging to continue with a diet if you feel it has not done you any good after a while. There is a way to get around this discouragement, however, and it is super simple.

Take a full body picture of yourself. Save it, and save the outfit you were wearing that day. This will be your before picture used for later comparison. Once you see the difference in person, it changes things and makes it easier to continue.

After you take your before photo, take another photo one week later. Wear the same outfit, so you can really tell a difference without the interference of how varying outfits make you look. The first week picture may not look a lot different, but don't be discouraged, sustainable and healthy weight loss should not be fast-tracked.

Start taking a picture every week in the same outfit, and standing in the same positions with both side and frontal view. You will begin to see a difference in the pictures gradually, and that makes everything worth it.

You can also track your weight loss, but do not get hung up on this part. Weight is only part of a diet and easily occluded by factors such as water retention or daily digestion. If you are exercising, it may not be pounds that start dropping initially, it will probably be inches off your waist. Your weight may even go up a few pounds or so as your fat stores are being turned into muscle.

However, if you feel you have to weigh yourself, do not do so more than once every week. Take off your shoes, and weigh yourself on the same day to remain consistent. You will see a gradual, fluctuating change in your weight, and this can be a great thing to see.

You can also track inches off your waist. This is the most solid type of weight loss tracking. You can literally see the unwanted fat disappearing. This is highly motivating, as the more progress you see, the more drive you have to align to flexible dieting and it will allow you to see greater progress in the weeks to come.

Eating Out on a Flexible Diet

One of the perks of this diet is that it allows you to eat out at any restaurant. You don't have to order only low carb menu options, or just a salad, either. You can eat the regular food that is there and not have to worry about having a cheat day. Just try to fit it into your macros.

To do this, often times you need to cut down the portion of what you eat. Restaurants frequently serve more than the healthy portion, and we try to eat it all. This is not what should be done. Instead, fill up mainly on water, and then eat half of what you are brought. Take the other half home for lunch tomorrow. By cutting down your portion, you ensure that you will still be in the confines of your macros without going over, or using up too many of your macros so you can't eat much more that day.

Enjoy the food you eat. Don't pick something you don't really like just because you are scared to go over your macros. The whole point of IIFYM is to not feel like you are on a diet, and to be able to eat the foods you love. Go out and indulge in your cravings, just remember not to binge eat it.

Mistakes to Avoid

While this diet is easy, there are still some mistakes you should try to avoid, as they can cause you to lose focus and commitment to IIFYM. These mistakes are pretty easy to overcome if you know what to look for. It just takes a little bit of patience and a lot of will power.

- When you think of your favorite food, do you think moderation? No? That is where the first mistake comes in. Most people eat all they want of their favorite foods, and then run out of macros by the time the day is half over, so they have to either go over their macros, or be hungry for the rest of the day. This is one of the biggest mistakes that people make in this diet. They think flexible diet means eat all they want as long as they exercise. But in reality this diet is still a diet. While you don't have to limit yourself in terms of what you can eat, you do have to limit yourself in the terms of how much you can eat. You can't pig out on donuts all day and expect to lose weight.

- Another mistake is being overly cautious with your macros. When you are too cautious and don't eat much during the day, you have to make up for it at night. This is a bad idea, because at night, your body is beginning to get ready for bed and slows down your metabolism. This means that your food will not be broken down as efficiently. So if you consume a big meal to try to make your macros limit at the last minute, then you are bogging down your metabolism, and this can actually cause weight gain rather than weight loss. Eat well, and if you don't quite make it to your goal, it is better to be just under, than to try to cram it all in one meal.

- IIFYM is not an excuse for you to live off of junk food, while saying you are on a diet. For optimal health and performance, don't use flexible dieting as an excuse to skip veggies in favor of sweets. Make the conscious decision to incorporate a variety of nutrient-dense foods such as fruits, vegetables and wholegrain sources of carbs. You should still eat healthy food. Put away the snack cakes and pick up a homemade muffin. If you consume mainly junk food, your trans fat levels are going to be excessive, and that will cancel out any of the good fats you have consumed, making you sluggish and tired, so you will be unable to exercise, and then you will just gain a lot of weight.

- Don't go into this diet with a poor mindset. This sets you up for failure immediately. If you are skeptical, get someone to try it with you so that you can be sure it will work and that you will stick with it. Go into this diet with the mindset that by the time it is done, you will have the body you always dreamed of.

- How many times have you tried to diet, made a mistake, and then gave up? This is another mistake that many of the dieters make. Even on this diet. One cheat day isn't going to ruin your whole diet. If you mess up, just try again. There is no need to give up. Was Rome built in a day? No. It takes time for these things to become a second nature to you. Until that point, mistakes will happen.

- Diets are not always a walk in the park. There are many different mistakes that you can make that can derail your progress. Don't let them completely destroy all of your progress. Because if you let them do that, all your hard work is for nothing. If you mess up, sit back and figure out where exactly you went wrong, and what steps you are going to take to avoid making the same mistake again. Then once you figure that out, it is time to try again. Continue doing this until you have all the flaws worked out and form strategies to minimize future mistakes.

- I am sure you have heard all of the things that people say to sway others against the norm. Those with negative or pessimistic mindsets will try to do the same to you, because you get to enjoy your diet, while they are still stuck on having to restrict themselves. This will make them bitter, and they may try to make you miserable as well. Don't let them. Show them how well it works, and get them out of your ear. Listening to these words would be the biggest mistake you could ever make, because you miss out on one of the world's simplest diets. If you listen to them, you will not be in the right mindset to achieve the body you want. The only way to validate their words is to let them get to you. If you stay above them, they can't bring you down.

Bonus Tips

There are a few extra things you should know about flexible dieting. These tips are all optional, but give you an extra boost to success. Utilize these mini goals throughout your dieting phase and they will help you become the best you that you can be.

- The first tip is to enlist the help of a buddy. Find a friend who also is burnt out on regular diets and wants to try something new, and see if he or she would like to try this diet with you. When you have a friend it makes it a lot easier to stick with something. You have someone to exercise with, and someone to share ideas with and be accountable to. Also you have someone to eat with when you want to try something new. Do not underestimate companionship as a powerful motivator.

- Gather a great support system. This is not like enlisting a friend into the diet. Your support system does not have to follow the diet to support you. They just have to believe in you so that you can push through, and meet your goals. It is always nice to have someone rooting for you as you push towards the finish line. If you have a great group of people behind you, then you can't fail, because they won't allow you to. Family members, work colleagues, or peers are people you can engage in this regard. Share your goals and be open to their feedback.

- Find a good gym and an even better exercise program. Part of making any diet successful is physical activity. The more energy you expend, the more food is getting used up in your system, and the healthier your body is. You work your body and the muscles in your heart, and that makes for a great overall wellbeing, both physically and psychologically. You don't have to become a bodybuilder, just find a routine that has a nice balance of cardio and weight work. Also do not discount the value of incidental exercise. Take the stairs, stretch at your desk, walk to the shops, it all adds up. Exercise will boost your weight loss beyond that of flexible dieting alone.

- Don't fall for placebos. There is no miracle weight loss pill or supplement out there that will make you lose an exorbitant amount of weight in a short timeframe. Avoid pricey strict diet and exercise plans, the internet is full of free high quality resources if you research properly. YouTube is also a great resource for sourcing information and workouts to follow, as well as additional IIFYM guidance. Don't waste your money, and just follow the diet itself.

You can do this, and if you ever get discouraged, just come back to this book. I believe in you. This may just be words on a page, but you can do it. You have it in you to make it through this, and become a healthy person, and get the body and lifestyle you DESERVE. Go get 'em!!

Conclusion

Thank you again for taking the time to read this book. I hope that you found it educational and inspiring. Macros are a very important part of a healthy flexible diet, and I hope now you see that and will apply what you learned in this book to your habits in real life.

Best of luck on your weight loss journey, and I know that you will make your goal. I hope that you use this book as a boost to get there and refer back to it often.

About The Author

Connor Harper

With a background in Exercise Physiology, Connor has been working as a personal trainer and coach for the past 10 years. His passion for research based methodology, customized approaches to fit client needs, and embedding fitness as a way of life, has made his coaching programs highly coveted in the industry. He has worked successfully with a variety of people, from stay at home mums to award winning body builders.

Connor believes that anyone can build on their strength and conditioning, regardless of starting point. He continues to encourage others to reap the benefits of having an active lifestyle.

He lives in Houston, Texas, with his wife and little girl. In his spare time, he loves to cook hearty meals for his family and train in Brazilian Jiu Jitzu.

Stay connected to Connor's future publications at www.bookwormhaven.com

Made in the USA
Middletown, DE
18 July 2018